THE POCKET GUIDE TO CRITICAL APPRAISAL

THE POCKET GUIDE TO CRITICAL APPRAISAL: A HANDBOOK FOR HEALTH CARE PROFESSIONALS

by
IAIN K. CROMBIE

*Department of Epidemiology & Public Health,
Ninewells Hospital & Medical School, Dundee, Scotland*

© BMJ Publishing Group 1996

First published in 1996
Second impression 1997
by the BMJ Publishing Group, BMA House, Tavistock Square,
London WC1H 9JR

British Library Cataloguing in Publication Data

A catalogue record for this book is available from the British Library

ISBN 0-7279-1099-X

Typeset by Apek Typesetters Ltd, Nailsea, Bristol
Printed and bound in Great Britain by Latimer Trend Ltd, Plymouth

Contents

Preface

This book was written to meet the needs of health professionals as medicine moves to be evidence-based. The initial idea arose during discussion with postgraduate students on their difficulties of interpreting the medical literature. It quickly became apparent that their needs would be best met by a short book detailing criteria for critical appraisal.

The book is organised in two parts. The first five chapters provide an introduction to critical appraisal, indicating how papers can be read and how the results can be interpreted. Experienced researchers could easily omit these chapters. The final six chapters provide annotated check lists for critical appraisal. The first of these contains the general questions which can be asked of any study, irrespective of the method used. The succeeding chapters review, in turn, the questions which are specific for each research method. For convenience, each of the latter chapters concludes with a combined list of general and specific questions.

The book has been written to be simple to use. Technical terms are avoided where possible, and the assessment criteria are explained but not justified. A larger and less accessible text would have been needed to give a proper rationale for each of the check lists. To keep this a pocket guide it was also decided to omit evaluations of other topics such as qualitative methods, health economics, clinical audit, decision analysis, and screening tests. An argument could be made for the inclusion of each, but to include them all would nearly double the size of the book. I hope the check lists provided prove useful.

I K CROMBIE

Acknowledgements

I was encouraged to write this book by my colleague and friend Huw Davies. Several other colleagues gave constructive comments on the manuscript, including Fiona Williams, Linda Irvine, Beth Alder, Gordon McLaren, Jane Knight, and Charles Florey. Special thanks go to Janet Tucker whose gentle but incisive comment "it won't work that way" led to a substantial improvement in the text. The check lists were based on my own experiences of conducting research and refereeing papers, but I have augmented and improved them through comparison with previously published ones. I gratefully acknowledge my debt to the authors of these check lists. The preparation of this book was supported by the Scottish Office Home and Health Department.

1 Introducing critical appraisal

The medical literature is vast and rapidly expanding. Forays into the library can be exhausting, as the reader is overwhelmed by the papers on offer. When read, some will cite interesting references which spur the reader into a lengthy paper chase. A major hazard of reading is to pursue a subject in too much depth. Instead of following this haphazard course, the process of reading should be carefully planned to provide a worthwhile return on the time invested. Establishing control over your reading means following a number of steps:

- Clarify your reasons for reading
- Specify your information need
- Identify the relevant reports
- Critically appraise the papers.

Clarify your reasons for reading

Health professionals read the literature for many reasons: to keep up to date, to answer specific clinical questions, or to pursue a research interest. Each reason requires a different kind of literature search. To keep abreast of professional developments a skim through the most recent issues of the main journals will suffice. Specific clinical questions can be answered by reading recent high quality studies. In contrast, pursuing a research interest can require an extensive computerised literature search to determine whether the study has been done before. Whatever the reason for reading, the library should be approached only when the reasons for reading have been clarified.

Specify your information need

Clarifying what you want to find out should indicate the amount of information required. Many queries can be best answered from current textbooks or review articles. But these will not contain the most recent studies, and will not contain the level of detail of the original papers. Thus, the reader should ask: What kind of reports do I want? How much detail do I need? How comprehensive do I need to be? How far back should I search? The answers to these questions follow from the reasons for reading.

Identify the relevant reports

Knowing what you want to find out leads to the question of how to get it most easily. There are many ways of accessing the literature in addition to browsing through journals: indexing journals such as *Index Medicus*; abstracting journals like *Current Contents*; computerised literature searches using Medline. The local librarian will advise on the types of search which you can conduct. There are usually several ways of tracking down papers, so any library search should be approached by asking how this can be done most easily.

Even brief visits to the library can generate several dozen papers to inspect. Many will be of marginal relevance, and should be set aside. Selectivity in reading is essential to ensure that there is time for the detailed inspection of important papers.

Critically appraise the papers

Having identified potentially useful articles, they need to be appraised critically. The process of appraisal is the focus of this book. There are many poor quality studies whose claims should be discounted. Others contain some information of value mixed in with much that is dross. This book provides check lists by which the useful information can be readily identified.

2 Questions to ask when reading a paper

Research papers are organised into four main sections: introduction, methods, results, and discussion. Most also begin with an abstract or summary which presents the key points from each of the main sections. Papers can be read by asking a series of questions, addressed to the various sections. These questions will elicit the important information that each section contains, and will also provide the basis for the evaluation of the quality of the study. The questions are:

- Is it of interest?
- Why was it done?
- How was it done?
- What has it found?
- What are the implications?
- What else is of interest?

Is it of interest? Title, abstract

An immediate guide to whether a paper may be worth reading comes from the title and abstract. This will indicate how relevant the topic is to the information needed and how interesting the results are likely to prove. The abstract should also give a preliminary indication of how well the study was conducted.

Why was it done? Introduction

The main function of the introduction is to provide the background to the study, indicating why it was carried out. To do this the introduction briefly reviews previous work, but does so mainly to highlight gaps in our current knowledge. It can also show why these are major gaps which urgently need to be filled. Often this is achieved by describing the clinical importance of the topic in terms of mortality, morbidity, or cost to the health service.

The introduction should end with a clear statement of the purpose of the study. This may be phrased as a hypothesis to be tested or as a question to be answered. The absence of such a statement can imply that the authors themselves had no clear idea of what they were trying to find out. If this were the case it is likely that they did not find out much of interest.

How was it done? Methods

The methods section gives the details of how the study was carried out. The descriptions are usually succinct, and references are often given to papers which provide fuller explanations. Despite this brevity, there should be sufficient information to indicate who was studied and how they were recruited (for example, which clinic the patients attended, what the diagnostic criteria were, what age and sex groups were included). Without this information it will not be possible to say how widely the findings can be generalised.

There should also be sufficient detail to allow the reader to decide whether the data which have been collected are accurate. If measurements were made, the circumstances in which they were taken should be described, together with the steps taken to standardise the measuring procedures. The structure of any questionnaires used should also be given, and mention made of how they were tested for validity and reliability. The information in the methods section provides an important guide to the quality of the paper. Finally, the methods section should indicate which statistical methods were used in the analysis.

What has it found? Results

The main findings of the study are presented in tables and figures which are explained by the text in the results section. The data should be presented in a logical fashion, starting with quite simple observations and proceeding, when appropriate, to complex analyses. The text should lead the reader through the data, highlighting the key findings. When the results follow a more haphazard course, which impedes understanding, they may not have been fully analysed.

The text in the results section will give the author's view of what is important. This need not be the only view; authors can make mistakes. Readers should make up their own minds about what the study has found. It is also worth checking whether the results fulfil the aims of the study. When an aim presented in the introduction is not addressed in the results, a number of questions arise. Why was it missed? Was this just an oversight? Were the appropriate data not collected? Or were the findings, for some reason, unacceptable to the authors? The omission raises doubts about the whole paper.

Another warning sign is when the paper does not expand on phrases like: "the results for the analysis are shown in Table 2". This can suggest that the authors have not worked out what the findings really mean. If they do not have the interest to interpret their own data they may not have had the application to design and conduct the study properly.

As part of the interpretation of the results the reader should search for the flaws and inconsistencies in the study. All research is flawed in some way, and it is simply a matter of finding out how. Often the problems are minor and can be ignored, but sometimes they may undermine the main findings. Critical appraisal does not just involve *finding* flaws; their potential impact must also be assessed. Only then can a decision be made on what the results really mean.

What are the implications? Abstract/discussion

The value of research usually lies in the extent to which the findings can be generalised to other times and other locations. A study which has meaning only for the clinic in which it was conducted is almost certainly not worth reading. The wider implications of a study should be reviewed in the discussion, and they are often summarised in the abstract.

Identifying implications is largely a subjective process, and as such should be approached with caution. We would all like our own studies to have earth-shaking significance. Thus it is not surprising that authors are not always impartial when interpreting their results. The following questions should be asked when assessing the implications: What is new? What does it mean for health care? Is it relevant to my patients? Certainly the findings should be compared with other studies and any discrepancies addressed. The key question for health professionals is whether the findings should be acted upon by introducing changes in current clinical practice.

The answer is best delayed until the check lists presented in Chapters 6 to 11 have been scrutinised.

What else is of interest? Introduction/discussion

The results contained in a paper may not be the only interesting feature. Useful references may be cited in the introduction and discussion. These sections may also discuss important or novel ideas. Thus, even if the results are to be discounted, there may still be benefit to reading a paper. Critical appraisal is not just a fault-finding exercise. It is a process of reviewing a paper to identify information of value.

3 Identifying the research method

Many of the criteria for appraisal apply to all methods of research. But others are specific to a single method. Thus, the use of the detailed check lists requires first that the research method be identified. This chapter provides an outline of the research methods to be used for identification. It does not attempt to provide a definitive description of each method as this would entail much more detail than is needed. Instead, it just gives sufficient detail to enable the reader to recognise one when it is used.

There are several key terms which are specific for certain methods; technically, they should be diagnostic for the method. Unfortunately some authors use these terms indiscriminately so that their appearance in the text does not necessarily identify the method. There is no recourse but to look in detail at how the study was conducted to confirm the method used. In most instances this will be a simple matter, with difficulties arising only when the authors misuse key terms.

Surveys

Surveys are used to describe how things are now. A sample of individuals is identified, and data are obtained on each at more or less the same time. The sample being studied may be taken from the general population, or may be a highly selected one. For example, surveys could be carried out to establish the levels of serum cholesterol in the general population. However, surveys can also be used to study specific groups such as pregnant women, physiotherapists, or persons aged between 65 and 90 years. Surveys can even be carried out on inanimate objects such as fire extinguishers, or emergency trolleys.

Essential features

In principle, surveys start by obtaining a complete list of the group of interest. Then a sample of individuals on the list is selected for further study. The selection is carried out randomly (not haphazardly) so that each individual has an equal chance of being chosen. In practice, a complete list of the group may not be available, and imaginative alternative methods may be used. However, the overall process should achieve the same end: random sampling should be used to obtain a representative sample. Data are then collected on the current status of the sampled individuals.

Complications

Most surveys do not have a separate control or comparison group. Thus, studies which have them are usually not surveys. However, in the analysis of surveys one subgroup in the sample may be compared with another (for example, men versus women, or old versus young). Comparisons are being made but there is no sense in which one group is acting as a control to another group. All the individuals have been selected at the same time and then internal comparisons are made.

Terms of identification

Use of the term *survey* in a paper should identify the method, but sometimes the term is mistakenly used for what is really a cohort study. *Cross-sectional* is a helpful term because it is seldom used with any other research method. The terms *sample* and *random sample* are unhelpful because they often appear in the description of the other research designs. There are many different ways of drawing a sample, described by the terms *stratified, cluster,* and *systematic.* These terms are seldom used with the other research methods, except stratified, which can be used in a clinical trial.

Cohort studies

Cohort studies are used to find out what happens to patients. For example, they could investigate how long patients with acute low-back pain take to recover; or they could monitor the natural history of peptic ulcers. Whatever the topic, a group of individuals is identified and watched to see what events befall them. Cohort studies may have a comparison or control group. These will be identified at about the same time and will be followed for roughly the same length of time. However, a control group is not an essential feature, and many cohort studies do not have one.

Essential features

The defining characteristic of cohort studies is the element of time: in cohort studies time flows forwards. A set of individuals is identified at one point in time, and followed up to a later time to ascertain what has happened. The direction of time is always forwards. Studies in which individuals are selected at one point and traced backwards to see how they were at some time previously are not cohort studies.

Complications

Cohort studies can be readily imagined as identifying a group of patients and following them into the future. However, some studies identify a set of patients at some time in the past and follow them up to the present. These studies might at first appear to be looking backwards in time, but they are not. Time flows forwards from the point at which the patients are identified.

Terms of identification

The term *cohort* should be diagnostic for this method, although sometimes the word is used in the context of clinical trials. The same counsel applies to the terms *prospective, follow-up,* and *outcome.* The term *retrospective* can be used of cohort studies which have identified a set of patients at some time in the past. However, this term is also used with case–control studies.

Clinical trials

Clinical trials should be the easiest method to identify. They are used to test whether one health care intervention is superior to another. Clinical trials are often described in terms of testing drugs, but they can be used to investigate many different types of health care intervention: surgery, vaccination, anti-pressure sore mattresses, and health education. When a completely new type of treatment has been developed it may be tested against a placebo because there is no other treatment to compare it against.

Essential features

Clinical trials are always concerned with effectiveness. A characteristic of well-conducted clinical trials is that they identify a set of patients with a diagnosed disease, and then randomly allocate them to the new or current best treatment. The focus of the study should be on the outcome of the treatments, seeking the one which is superior. Clinical trials are also concerned with the side-effects of treatments.

Complications

Sometimes cohort studies are used to assess effectiveness; in such studies a group of treated patients is followed up to see how many gain benefit. Cohort studies are a poor method of assessing a treatment and can be severely criticised: it is difficult to make a fair comparison between treatments in a cohort study.

The brief outline of clinical trials stated that two treatments were being compared. This is commonly the case, but in some instances more than two treatments can be investigated. Doing so adds to the complexity of the study and its analysis, although the resulting study can still be a valid clinical trial.

Terms of identification

The terms *effectiveness, efficacy,* and *evaluation* or phrases like *assess the value of* or *improve the outcome*, are often used in papers on clinical trials. The terms *double blind* and *placebo-controlled* are seldom used except in a clinical trial. *Random allocation* of patients to treatments is essential for a fair comparison, and thus its presence suggests that a study is a clinical trial. (However, the term *random selection* is more likely to refer to a survey.) The simple term *outcome* can feature in cohort studies as well as in clinical trials.

Case–control studies

Case–control studies ask what makes a group of individuals different. Often the group of individuals will have some disease, in which case the question will be directed at the causes of their disease. In other instances the individuals will have behaved in some way, such as failed to comply with therapy or failed to attend for a clinic appointment.

Essential features

Case–control studies select a set of patients with a defining characteristic: a diagnosed disease (for example, women with breast cancer) or lack of attendance at breast screening. The characteristics of these are compared with a control group (often similar in age, sex, and background) who do not have the characteristic of interest.

Complications

Case–control studies often have an element of time in which a backwards look is taken to past events. They look to see whether current disease could have been caused by past events. The directionality of time is crucial for distinguishing between cohort studies and case–control studies: cohorts look forwards, case–control studies look backwards.

Terms of identification

As well as *case–control* there are several other terms for this type of study, including *case–referrent, case–comparator* and *case–comparison*. The possession of a control group is not a defining characteristic because clinical trials should also have one, and cohort studies often do. Because the method looks backwards in time it is sometimes called a *retrospective study*, but this term can be used for cohort studies.

4 Interpreting the results

Interpreting the results presented in a paper provides the major challenge to the critical faculties. Each table and figure should be approached asking "what do I think this really means?". Caution is the watchword: large, exciting and unexpected results are exceedingly rare. In contrast, flawed studies and misleading findings are much more common. Results should be approached with care by assessing their significance and by looking for possible pitfalls in the analysis. This chapter presents fundamental ideas for the interpretation of results.

Statistical significance

In the past some papers simply presented tables and graphs with a description and explanation of the main findings. It is now conventional for research studies to assess the statistical significance of the findings through statistical tests. The need for statistical tests arises because of the pervasiveness of the play of chance.

The play of chance

Whenever a group of patients is selected for study, and measurements are made, there is an opportunity for the play of chance to affect the findings. The effects of chance are most evident with small samples. Suppose a sample of ten newborn babies was taken. Although we would expect that about half would be girls, no one would be surprised if there were seven girls and only three boys. If a second sample were taken, the observation of four girls and six boys would, again, cause no concern. Although in the long run we expect approximately equal numbers of boys and girls, the play of chance means that we seldom get a 50:50 split in small samples.

The effects of the play of chance are seen everywhere in medical research. Suppose two treatments are being compared in a clinical trial. Patients will have been randomly allocated to the two groups. Randomisation protects against systematic differences between the two groups, but it does not prevent differences arising by chance. For example, it could happen that slightly more of the severely ill patients could have been allocated to one treatment group, creating an apparent difference between the treatments even if there were none. In practice it is very unusual for the two groups in a clinical trial to be exactly the same: there are often small chance differences between them. Less often, there are very large chance differences between the two groups.

The importance of the play of chance lies in the extent to which it might have affected the observed results. Sometimes, what looks like an interesting result may finally prove to be a statistical fluke. Fortunately, statistical methods allow us to estimate whether or not the observed results could be due to the play of chance. Central to these methods is the concept of probability.

Probability

The probability of throwing a six (with a fair, six-sided dice) is one in six. The probability of a single ticket winning the national lottery is one in 14 million. Probabilities are simply a way of describing how likely it is that an event will happen. They are often expressed as decimal fractions, where one in six becomes 0·167. The interpretation of probabilities is quite straightforward. When an event has a very small probability, for example, 0·0001, it is very unlikely to happen. When the probability is large, say 0·9, the event is very likely to happen.

Probabilities vary between 0·0 and 1·0, where zero means an event will never happen and 1·0 means it is certain to happen. Thus, the probability that a healthy adult will eventually die is 1·0, because we all die sometime. In contrast, the probability of the adult dying tomorrow is less than one in 100 000, i.e. 0·00001. It is not quite zero because some unlikely event, such as being run over by a bus, might just happen. But it is very small because unlikely events are unlikely to happen.

Probabilities lie at the heart of statistical tests. They are often termed P-values, in which the letter P stands for probability. They

13

can be written as $P = 0.003$, indicating that an event has a three in 1000 chance of occurring, a somewhat rare occurrence. Sometimes this will be written $P < 0.01$, where the "<" symbol means "less than". The decimal 0.003 is less than 0.01, so if $P = 0.003$ it is also true that P will be less than 0.01. The "<" symbol is widely used, but saying $P < 0.01$ is less accurate than $P = 0.003$. There was a fashion for using the "<" symbol, where probabilities were rounded up to certain values. The most common were $P < 0.05$, $P < 0.01$, and $P < 0.001$. However, it is now preferred to give the exact P value because rounding up leads to an approximate value which wastes information.

The logic of statistical tests

Statistical tests use what sometimes appears to be a curious logic. It can seem that they do so just to be difficult, but the approach is chosen because it is the only one which is valid. Consider a study comparing two treatments in a clinical trial in which one treatment gives better results than the other. The first step is to propose that the difference observed between the treatments is due solely to the play of chance, i.e. that there is really no difference between the treatments. (This is not what we are hoping for: everyone would want a new treatment to be superior to the conventional one. However, it is the way the logic leads us.) The statistical test then calculates how likely it was that, by chance alone, we would have seen a difference at least as big as that observed. The test provides us with a probability, a P value, of the results being due to chance. When this is very small (for example, $P < 0.001$), we conclude that the result is unlikely to be due to chance. This leads us to reject the proposal that there is no difference between the treatments; we can conclude that one really is better than the other. (The hypothesis that there is no difference between the two treatments, other than that due to chance, is commonly called the *null hypothesis*.)

The P-value is a very convenient guide to whether or not the observed results could be due to chance: small P-values indicate that the result is unlikely to be due to chance. All we have to decide is when the P-value is small enough. There is a convenient, if arbitrary, rule: when the P-value is less than 0.05 (i.e. $P < 0.05$) we exclude chance as an explanation. When the P-value is this small the result is said to have achieved statistical significance.

The arbitrary rule ($P < 0.05$) does not correspond to a guarantee. Suppose we carried out a large number of statistical tests. We would expect a spuriously significant result to occur on average once for every 20 significance tests which have been carried out. (This is because $P = 0.05$ actually says that the chance alone could create the result one time in 20.) There are two corollaries. First, studies which have conducted a multitude of significance tests will regularly encounter spuriously significant results. Second, smaller P-values, say $P < 0.01$ or even $P < 0.001$, give increased confidence that the result was not a chance affair.

Confidence intervals

Confidence intervals provide an alternative way of assessing the effects of chance. They can also be more informative. Suppose a clinical trial of two antihypertensive drugs showed that one lowered diastolic blood pressure by an average of 15 mm Hg, whereas a second lowered it by an average of only 5 mm Hg. The average difference of 10 mm Hg seems impressive, but we know that this value could be influenced by chance. The important question is whether the true value for the difference between treatments could be as low as zero (i.e. no difference). We can tell this from the 95% confidence interval. It gives the range within which we are 95% certain that the true value lies. If the antihypertensive trial had given a range of 3 to 17, we would say that the true value could be as low as 3 or as high as 17. Zero lies outside this interval so we conclude that it is unlikely to be the true value. This is equivalent to obtaining a P-value of $P < 0.05$, i.e. the result achieved statistical significance. (Note that if the confidence interval had been wider, say ranging from -4 to 24, the interpretation would be different. This range includes zero, so that it could be the true value. We would then conclude that we have no evidence that there is a difference between the treatments.)

Confidence intervals are always interpreted in the same way, whether the research method was a clinical trial, a cohort study, or whatever. They are inspected to test the proposal that there was no effect, for example, no difference between two groups. If the zero difference lies within the confidence interval we conclude that there was no effect. If it lies outside the range, we exclude no effect as being unlikely. This is equivalent to saying that the result was statistically significant.

The advantage of confidence intervals is that they do more than indicate whether the result might be a chance effect. They show, allowing for the play of chance, how small and how large the true size of effect might be.

Pitfalls in the analysis

P-values and confidence intervals provide a valuable guide to the interpretation of results when the analysis has been carried out correctly. But there is the challenge of identifying when the analysis is flawed. From the details given in a paper it can be difficult to tell whether there are flaws in the analysis. All statistical tests make some assumptions about the data, but without access to the raw data it is not possible to test whether they have been met. Nonetheless, there are some pointers to possible defects.

Outliers

When data are presented in tables and figures there is the opportunity to look for outliers. An outlier is an unusually high or low value. For example, most of the values for the diastolic blood pressure of adults in the general population would be expected to lie between 65 and 90 mm Hg. Data points as low as 40 or as high as 130 mm Hg would be termed outliers. They may be correct values, or they may have been incorrectly recorded. The occurrence of a few observations which lie apart from the bulk of the data can distort the results. Their effect is similar to that seen with a see-saw which is very long on one side and conventionally short on the other. A small child placed on the long arm can overcome the weight of a much heavier child on the short arm. In statistical tests a few distant points can pull against the bulk of the data, creating misleading effects. There is no general rule for dealing with outliers, but if they are present some steps should be taken to investigate their effects. Ignoring outliers casts doubt on the whole of the analysis; instead, the paper should describe how they were coped with.

Skew

Some measurements, such as length of in-patient stay, tend to be grouped around an average value but with a long tail of high values. The high values can't be called outliers because they are not really separate from the bulk of the data. Instead, they gradually shade away from the most common values. The presence of a long tail of observations on one side of the average is called skewness. Skew acts in the same way as outliers to distort statistical tests. It is commonly seen when the observations involve time – for example, waiting times in clinics, or survival times of cancer patients. Sometimes allowance can be made for the presence of skew by transforming the data, for example, taking logarithms of the values to pull in the high ones. If there is evidence of skewness some explanation, often in the methods section, should be given about how it was coped with.

Non-independence

A common assumption in statistical tests is that all the observations are independent. For example, if a survey was measuring the heights of a sample of schoolchildren it would be assumed that measuring the height of one child would have no effect on the measurement of the next child. The assumption that all the measurements are independent could be breached if some of the children were measured more than once. There are special statistical methods (repeated measures designs) which can cope with this problem. But most of the common statistical tests cannot. In some studies some individuals are measured several times to try to increase the sample size. This is valid only when the statistical methods can take account of the non-independence of the data.

Serendipity masquerading as hypothesis

Many, if not most, research studies collect quite large amounts of data on the subjects being studied. These studies may have been set up to test a few specific hypotheses. However, there are usually many other avenues which can be explored: the relationship between the variables; the effects seen when the data are subdivided (for example, by age, sex, or severity of disease). Such detailed investigation is quite valid; indeed, it would be wasteful not to explore the data fully. Where things start to go wrong is when chance observations are presented as if they were hypotheses which were being tested. For example, in a clinical trial of two antihypertensives, the researchers might check whether the same size of effect was seen in the young compared with the old, or in men compared with women. It would be legitimate to report any difference seen between these subgroups. But, unless it had been clearly specified in advance of the analysis, it would be wrong to pretend that this was a hypothesis that the study was set up to test. There are many ways in which the data can be subdivided, so that by chance alone some are going to reveal apparently interesting effects. Subgroup analyses can generate lots of interesting observations which can then be tested in subsequent studies. A single set of data cannot be used to generate and test hypotheses.

Black-box analyses

Appropriate statistical tests increase the credibility of a paper. However, it does not follow that the more sophisticated the tests used the more authoritative the findings. Present day computer packages make it very easy to carry out complex analyses, even when the user has an incomplete understanding of the method being used. The more complex analyses tend to make more assumptions about the data being analysed. It is also much easier to make mistakes during the analysis.

Papers which present only the results of some complex analysis should be viewed with some suspicion. This approach makes it more difficult to identify problems in the data, such as skewness and outliers. It is better if the results of more simple analyses are presented first. Then these can be checked to see whether they accord with the more complex. If discrepancies are found they should be explained in the text of the paper. Unexplained discrepancies cast doubt on the propriety of the analysis.

Bias

Bias is the bugbear of research. It means that the results we get are systematically different from what they should have been. Bias can occur in a variety of guises but its effect is always the same: the observed results are misleading and the conclusions drawn may be wrong.

Bias can arise when the study subjects were selected. Even when the study has been carried out carefully, it is possible that those included differ from the general run of subjects. Some could have been included because they were more severely ill and hence, being bed-bound, were easily contacted. Alternatively, the severely ill might be excluded if, for example, they were away for treatment at a specialist centre. The need to obtain informed consent from the study subjects can also introduce bias. Those who refuse may differ from those who agree to co-operate. This problem is particularly acute for research concerned with attitudes and beliefs, as these are the very characteristics which influence participation in the study.

Bias can also occur when data are being collected. Measuring instruments may be wrongly calibrated, giving consistently high or low readings. The way in which questions are asked of patients may influence their replies: a sympathetic interviewer may encourage patients to describe their experiences in full. A second study with a more abrasive interviewer could gather much less detail, leading to the erroneous conclusion that there were changes in the patients' conditions. Misleading data can also be gathered when patients have to remember past events. Their recall may be influenced by many other factors, such as their need to find an explanation for their disease. Thus, a study of past events might be influenced more by factors affecting recall than by whether or not past events took place.

It is often difficult to determine whether bias has entered a study. The study methods need to be reviewed carefully. Having identified what was done, the question to be asked is: "how could it have gone wrong?". Playing devil's advocate by assuming that bias has occurred can assist in its identification.

Confounding

Confounding occurs when part of the observed relationship between two variables is due to the action of a third. For example, the consumption of alcohol will be related to lung cancer, but not because it causes this disease. Instead, both alcohol and lung cancer are related to smoking, and it is smoking which causes lung cancer.

Confounding arises because many aspects of human health and behaviour are interrelated. For example, with increasing age blood pressure tends to rise, and spectacles may be needed to help read the newspaper. This does not mean that hypertension causes hypermetropia. Instead, they reflect differing aspects of ageing. Thus, whenever a study shows that two factors are related, it should be asked whether a third factor could be driving the observed relationship.

5 Introduction to the check lists

The check lists provide a series of questions to be asked of published papers. The questions lead towards an informed judgement on the meaning of the findings and their relevance for clinical practice. Thus, the check lists provide a framework for the appraisal of papers. Each question has accompanying text which explains and expands on what is being assessed.

The check lists begin with a set of standard questions (Chapter 6) which apply irrespective of the research method which has been used. There follow five further check lists (Chapters 7 to 11) covering clinical trials, surveys, cohort studies, case–control studies, and review papers. These check lists are arranged in two parts. The first, the essential appraisal, acts as an initial screen to identify any major defects in the research. Thus, papers passing these checks have been given the equivalent of a provisional certificate of approval. Appraisal may stop at this stage, when the reader has identified a paper with potentially interesting new facts. However, if the paper is central to the reader's clinical practice then a more detailed assessment may be required. Equally, if a health professional is new to critical appraisal, then it will be helpful to review the second check list, the detailed appraisal.

The second check list provides for a more detailed review. It is organised in sections corresponding to the main sections of scientific papers. For convenience, the list incorporates the set of standard questions outlined in Chapter 6, but they are given in italics so that they can be easily distinguished. Together, the questions extend the process of uncovering and evaluating flaws in study design and execution. They also review the overall quality of the study and its analysis, and facilitate an assessment of the wider significance of the results. This simplifies the task of making a balanced assessment of the paper.

The complete check lists contain an extensive array of items for the assessment of published papers. However, these do not provide a tick-box guide to the quality of a paper. Many of the items require a subjective assessment of quality. In particular, flaws must be evaluated to determine their potential impact on the study findings.

Evaluating the flaws

Just because a study contains a flaw does not mean that it should be discarded. Given the difficulties of designing and conducting research, and the operation of Murphy's many laws of disaster, it is little surprise that many published papers contain flaws. Indeed, the dedicated critic could probably find some flaw in every paper. But many of these defects will be trivial, and will have almost no effect on the conclusions to be drawn from a study. Thus, the important question is not whether there are defects, but whether those defects matter. The flaws need to be evaluated to clarify which are serious and which are merely trivial.

It is difficult to draw up general rules for the evaluation of flaws because their impact will depend on the purposes of the study, the method employed, and the way the study was carried out. However, the items listed in the essential appraisal section specify the major flaws which can beset each type of method. If a study is seriously deficient on any of these it is quite likely that its conclusions are unfounded. For example, suppose a new drug for rheumatoid arthritis were being investigated. Treatments are best evaluated in randomised controlled trials. If the new drug had been tested in a study without a control group, any claims about effectiveness would be regarded with considerable scepticism.

As many flaws may have limited effect, simply counting their number can be unhelpful. A handful of minor flaws may have much less import than a single serious one. Instead, the flaws could be recorded along the lines indicated in Table 5.1. Writing these details can help to focus the mind and facilitate a decision on the merits of the paper.

Best case/worst case/likely case

Often it is difficult to judge what effect a defect may have on the study findings. A useful technique for many defects is to speculate

Table 5.1   Assessment of the importance of flaws

Flaws encountered	Type of flaw (nature and size)	Direction of effect	Is the finding of the study negated?
Design Conduct Interpretation			

on alternative possibilities, posing best case/worst case/likely case scenarios. Consider a postal questionnaire survey of the levels of literacy among elderly patients in long-term care. Suppose that it found that 90% had a high literacy score, but the response rate was only 50%. The low response rate could result in bias. The worst case would be that all the non-responders were illiterate, explaining why they did not reply. This would mean that the true proportion with a high literacy score was only 45%. Alternatively, it is possible that all the non-responders were highly literate, although this seems unlikely. The most likely case is that many non-responses occurred for reasons other than literacy, but that reading difficulties made a substantial contribution to the non-response. If it happened that half the non-response was due to poor literacy, then the true figure for high literacy would be 67·5%.

In practice we do not know the reasons for the 50% non-response but this type of speculation gives an indication of the consequences that bias could have. It will help to clarify whether the study results should be dismissed, or whether, with due caution, they can be accepted as an addition to our knowledge. For this example, given that the true level of high literacy could lie between 45% and 90%, the study findings would appear unreliable. Although the lower figure of 45% is unlikely to be correct, poor literacy is likely to make a substantial contribution to non-response. Thus, the study result of 90% is likely to be misleading. The size of effect of flaws should always be assessed to determine their likely impact on the study's conclusions.

6 The standard appraisal questions

There are several questions which should be asked of all research papers, irrespective of the method which has been used. These questions are described in this chapter. This set of questions is incorporated into the check lists provided in the following chapters, but the rationale for them is only given here. The questions follow the sequence in which information is presented in published papers:

Are the aims clearly stated?
Was the sample size justified?
Are the measurements likely to be valid and reliable?
Are the statistical methods described?
Did untoward events occur during the study?
Were the basic data adequately described?
Do the numbers add up?
Was the statistical significance assessed?
What do the main findings mean?
How are null findings interpreted?
Are important effects overlooked?
How do the results compare with previous reports?
What implications does the study have for your practice?

Are the aims clearly stated?

The aims of the study should be clearly stated, giving an explanation of why the study was carried out. This allows the reader to decide whether the research has tackled an important problem. Clearly stated and tightly focused aims suggest that the research hypothesis may have been specified in advance, resulting in a well planned study. In contrast, wide ranging or woolly aims suggest that many different issues were being pursued to see what popped up. Such studies are less likely to collect useful data. Further, they give the opportunity for trawling through the results, performing multiple significance tests. This makes it likely that some spurious statistically significant results would be obtained.

Was the sample size justified?

Research should be carried out only when it has a good chance of meeting the study aims. One essential part of this is that the study should be large enough to give an accurate picture of what is going on. Conventionally, the size of effect being sought (for example, the likely difference between two treatments) is specified. Then, a formal sample size calculation is carried out to determine how big the study should be to detect this effect. The details of this calculation should be in the methods section. Studies which are too small often fail to detect clinically important effects. When the trial has been completed, the question can be asked in a different form: what size of effect did the study have the power to detect? Studies of high quality address this issue, usually in the discussion section, but many studies ignore it.

Are the measurements likely to be valid and reliable?

Poor measuring techniques can lead to substantial errors. The methods of measurements should be described in some detail (references may be given to methods which are described elsewhere). They should be read critically, asking how errors could be introduced. Particular attention should be paid to difficult measurements, such as those involving subjective assessments. When there is more than one observer, for example in multicentre studies, some effort should have been made to standardise measurements. The issue of measurement error is often tackled in the discussion section, but if it is ignored the reader must ask whether there could be errors in measurement, and whether these could be important. The main concerns are whether the methods are likely to be valid and reliable.

A valid measure is one which measures what it is supposed to measure. For example, when estimating alcohol consumption, valid answers are unlikely to be obtained to the question "how much do you drink?". Many subjects will understate their true consumption, although some boastful ones may exaggerate. A reliable measure is one which gives a similar result when applied on more than one occasion. For example, in theory, an adult's height should be reliably measured, as it varies only slightly throughout the day. In practice, many factors, such as the way an individual stands, the way the measuring equipment is placed, whether or not shoes are worn, can contribute to differences between measurements. A feature of studies of high quality is that they discuss how validity and reliability were assessed.

Are the statistical methods described?

The statistical methods which were used should be described in the methods section, and should be referenced. Inappropriate statistical analysis can produce misleading results. All statistical tests make some assumptions about the data being analysed, and it is encouraging when this issue is explicitly addressed. If there is doubt about statistical propriety then it would be well to contact a statistician. One warning sign is the use of exotic statistical tests – was the test selected because of the P-value it yielded? Concern is heightened when the only results presented are those from a sophisticated statistical technique; simple analyses should be presented first and compared with the more complex ones. Another warning sign is the suggestion that a large number of tests were carried out – as more tests are carried out it becomes increasingly likely that spurious significance will result.

Did untoward events occur during the study?

In some studies it can prove difficult to follow exactly the initial research design, some subjects may not be contactable, and others may subsequently disappear. It may also prove impossible to make measurements on certain individuals. Most of these types of problem should have been identified and dealt with in pilot studies, so their occurrence in the main study may indicate inadequate preparation. Substantial amounts of missing data give ample opportunity for bias to intrude. More worrying is when problems encountered during the conduct of the study lead to changes in the design. Such changes may be poorly thought out and lead to further problems. For example, they could result in the data collected before the change being incompatible with those collected after. Some untoward events are truly unpredictable and

25

thus beyond the researcher's control, but often such events signal a study of poor quality.

Were the basic data adequately described?

All studies should report the number of subjects which were investigated, and how they were obtained. The basic characteristics of the subjects should be described, usually giving the mean or median for the principal measurements together with an indication of how the subjects vary (for example, the standard deviation or interquartile range). This information allows an assessment of the extent to which the findings can be generalised, and whether they are likely to be relevant to the reader's clinical practice.

The study should begin with sample analyses, giving the main outcomes in simple tables or figures. These give the reader a feel for what is going on in the data. Complex statistical methods which investigate the effects of many factors simultaneously, should be presented only after the simple analyses have been given. The findings from the more sophisticated analyses would normally fit with the more simple ones. Any discrepancy between these analyses should be explained in detail.

Do the numbers add up?

Subjects are sometimes lost from parts of a study, either because they truly disappeared, or because measurements made on them were not included in the final report. Many papers present several tables in which the data are subdivided in different ways. This provides an opportunity to check for absent subjects and missing data. Ideally, the number of subjects in all tables should add up to the value stated at the beginning of the results section (sometimes the number of subjects is given in the methods). Inconsistencies in the number of subjects should be explained in the text. Failure to do so indicates some sloppiness; the authors may not have checked the tables for typing errors, or they may be unconcerned about the consequences of missing data. Small discrepancies (of the order of 1%) are unlikely to have much impact on the findings, but large discrepancies are a serious hazard warning.

Was the statistical significance assessed?

The results of all research studies are influenced by the play of chance. Sometimes chance effects can appear quite large, especially when the sample size is small. Thus, the statistical significance of the main findings should be assessed. A P-value of less than 0·05 provides good evidence that the result is likely to be real rather than chance. Even smaller P-values, such as $P<0·01$, or $P<0·001$, give extra confidence that the result was not a chance event.

Many medical journals prefer confidence intervals to P-values. These also provide a test of statistical significance, but give additional information. They show the range within which the true value could lie (see Chapter 4). This allows an assessment of just how large, or how small, the true effect might be. Further, when the range is broad the meaning of the estimated size of effect is called into question.

What do the main findings mean?

The interpretation of study findings follows a standard sequence. The size of each reported effect is scrutinised to see whether it might be of clinical importance. The level of statistical significance is not necessarily a good guide to the clinical significance of a finding. However, the confidence interval can be helpful, showing the range within which the true value is likely to lie. The key findings can then be matched against any defects in the design, conduct and analysis, allowing the reader to make an informed decision about what the study has really shown. The author's conclusions cannot always be relied upon because researchers are often more enthusiastic about their findings than is strictly warranted. Instead, a careful search should be made for possible biases or confounding (see Chapter 4).

Findings can be given more weight when there is some internal consistency, i.e. similar results are seen when the data are divided into subgroups, such as age and sex. Supporting evidence, such as a dose–response relationship, also makes it more likely that the result is not a chance aberration (for example, that a moderate exposure carries a risk which is intermediate between low- and high-level exposures). Finally, the inherent plausibility of the results can be assessed. Do they make biological sense? Do they fit with what is known about the disease? Is the timing of the events plausible? The reader should not just accept the author's interpretation, but should mull over findings to decide whether, in their view, they make sense. Interpreting the findings of a study is a matter for judgement, aided by experience. The process may be subjective, and hence imperfect. But even an imperfect evaluation is better than passive acceptance of the results at face value.

How are null findings interpreted?

Null findings (for example, a new treatment which was found not to be better than a conventional one) need to be interpreted with particular care. The lack of an effect could arise because the study was too small to have a reasonable chance of detecting anything. This would be seen in the confidence interval, which would be wide. For example, in a clinical trial the confidence interval would cover a range from the new treatment being much better to the new treatment being much worse. Null findings can also arise through weaknesses in the design or conduct of the study. Whatever the explanation, lack of evidence of an association is not the same as evidence of no association.

Are important effects overlooked?

There is an understandable tendency among researchers to draw attention to findings which fit their preconceptions. Results which do not fit their views, or which flatly contradict them, are sometimes not commented on. Thus, the results need to be explored for interesting looking effects, even null findings, which are unremarked.

How do the results compare with previous reports?

The findings from a single study seldom provide convincing evidence. New findings are usually accepted only when there is a substantial body of research, involving several studies preferably from more than one research group. (Confidence is diminished if it is thought that other research groups have had difficulty in confirming a result.) Thus the results of any study need to be interpreted in the light of previous reports.

The supportive studies cited in a paper may not be sufficient to confirm a finding. Some authors may be tempted to overstate previous findings which support their own, and may omit mention of contradictory results. Instead, the findings from a single report need to be fitted into a balanced overview of all reported studies. This is seldom possible as only a small number of people will be expert in any given field. Nonetheless, the reader who is not familiar with a particular field should be more circumspect about accepting the claims of a single paper.

What implications does the study have for your practice?

Possibly the most important issue when reviewing a paper is whether it should lead to changes in the management of one's own patients. The decision can be between subjecting patients to useless therapy and denying them access to effective ones. Alternatively, it could be whether to advise them to avoid some harmful behaviour at the risk of generating anxiety. The first question is, how big was the effect, and is it clinically important? Then the quality of the study should be assessed, together with the amount of supporting evidence, asking whether the finding is likely to be true. Finally, the relevance of the finding to your practice should be reviewed by asking whether the patients studied were similar to yours and whether the conditions in which the study was carried out resemble local circumstances. This should indicate whether the same size of effect is likely to occur in your patients.

7 Appraising surveys

This chapter presents the issues which are relevant primarily to surveys. These are arranged in two parts: the brief essential questions and the more detailed specific questions. An explanation is given for each item. These lists are then combined, at the end of the chapter, with the list of standard questions described in Chapter 6. These lists provide a complete guide to the appraisal of surveys.

The essential questions

Surveys are easy to carry out. In consequence, the method is widely used and, some would say, widely abused. Surveys simply involve identifying a group of subjects – be they patients, health professionals, or members of the general population. Data are collected on each subject, often by questionnaire or interview. Surveys are used to make general statements about a group wider than that studied. It is the validity of these generalisations that lies at the heart of the brief appraisal of surveys.

Who was studied?
How was the sample obtained?
What was the response rate?

The specific questions

The specific questions are also concerned with the validity of the generalisations, but have a different focus. Their main concern is with the common pitfalls which beset the design and interpretation of surveys.

Is the design appropriate to the stated objectives?
Is there a suggestion of haste?
How could selection bias arise?
Were the findings serendipitous?
Can the results be generalised?

Rationale for the essential questions

Who was studied?

The interpretation of survey findings naturally depends on who is being investigated. The source of the sample will determine whether the results apply generally or whether they are restricted to a highly selected group. Selection criteria for entry into the sample (such as age, sex, or severity of disease) should be inspected carefully to see how these could influence the findings. A clear description of the source population allows an assessment of whether the method of drawing the sample is flawed.

How was the sample obtained?

The method of obtaining the sample is crucial to the validity of the findings. Some studies take what is called a grab sample of subjects. Individuals are included because they are convenient to hand, ignoring the problem that the factors which make them convenient may also make them unrepresentative. The personal case-series (for example, the patients treated at a particular clinic) falls into this category. It might be thought that the sample is comprehensive if all the patients seen over some time period are included. However, there are many selection factors that determine which patients are seen by a health professional: there will usually be many patients who do not make it through the gates controlling access to a clinic.

The process of obtaining a sample needs to be a rigorous one, and should be adequately described. Everyone who would be considered eligible for the study should have an equal chance of being selected for the sample. Thus, there needs to be some kind of list of all potential subjects, together with a mechanism for drawing a random sample (using random numbers). Sampling is flawed whenever there are groups of subjects who will be largely over-looked. The size of the problem will depend on the number overlooked, and the extent to which these subjects are likely to differ from those included.

What was the response rate?

In surveys, many subjects cannot be contacted, or refuse to take part. The concern with non-response is whether it could introduce bias. Those who do not respond often differ systematically from those who do. Individuals who have moved home or been admitted to long-term care, may be missed; those who have emigrated, or died, certainly will be. Information may also not be obtained on those who have difficulty reading, dislike filling in questionnaires (or taking part in interviews), or have some personal antipathy to the subject being investigated. The reasons which lead people to be difficult to contact also mark them out as being different from those contacted. Thus, once the study has been conducted it is worth asking "who is likely to be missed" and "what effect would this have on the results?".

The greater the percentage of non-responders, the larger the bias which could result. There is no magic rule for what is an acceptable response rate. Instead, the circumstances of the study should be reviewed, balancing the study findings against the size of non-response and the likely reasons for it. Best case/worst case calculations can be carried out (see Chapter 5). The question is to what extent have the findings been influenced by non-response? Studies which do not give the response rate, or claim a near-perfect response, should be regarded with suspicion. Unless the circumstances are quite exceptional, a captive audience who are compelled to answer, the response rate will always be less than 100%.

Rationale for the specific questions

Is the design appropriate to the stated objectives?

The evidence from surveys is considered particularly weak. Surveys can describe what is going on – for example, how care is currently being delivered, or whether patients were satisfied with their management. They can provide insight into the current organisation and consequences of care, but they are not well suited to explaining why events happen as they do. In particular, they cannot be used to assess whether one form of care was more effective than another. Surveys should be assessed by asking whether the study aims might be better met by one of the other research methods.

Is there a suggestion of haste?

A difficulty with surveys is that it is very easy to conduct one with only a vague idea of what is being investigated. There is a danger that they are undertaken before the details of the study design have been properly worked out. Thus, a few questions may be cobbled together and a questionnaire distributed to a set of individuals who are conveniently to hand.

Surveys which have been conducted in haste often give scant descriptions of how the sample was selected and how the measurements were made. Usually they will give no indication that a pilot study was carried out. Another warning sign is that no attempt has been made to contact those who did not respond to the first invitation to participate. The nature of the key findings should also be checked. If subtle or sensitive issues have been investigated then the methods section should explain how the questions were developed and tested. If physical measurements, such as height or blood pressure, have been taken then the steps taken to standardise the conditions of measurement should be described.

How could selection bias arise?

The possibility that the method of drawing the sample could affect the results was introduced in the brief appraisal questions. However, selection bias has such importance for surveys that it should be explicitly reviewed. The following questions are being asked: What could possibly happen to make atypical the sample that was obtained? Was the group from which the sample was drawn unusual in any way? Could the method of drawing the sample have introduced bias? Could certain types of participant have been selectively lost? Note that having a very large sample provides no protection. If selection bias is occurring it will have as great an effect on a study with one million participants as it would with one of 500.

Were the findings serendipitous?

Surveys provide the opportunity to collect data on many different items: the analysis then looks to see what falls out. Problems arise if unexpected results are presented as though they were the very findings which were being sought. This flawed procedure invalidates tests of statistical significance. If lots of data have been collected it is likely that several spurious statistically significant results will be found. Significance tests on survey data should be treated with great caution. They can be used as a method for discarding unimportant (i.e. non-significant) findings; the difficulty lies in interpreting the significant ones. Papers should be inspected carefully for suggestions that many statistical tests were carried out but that only the significant ones are presented.

Can the results be generalised?

The extent to which findings can be generalised, to other times and other locations, is of concern for all research methods. However, the issue is particularly acute for surveys because a sample has been taken precisely for what it says about some wider group. The extent of generalisation depends on how well the study performed on the other appraisal questions. If it appears robust, particularly on the essential questions, generalisations can be made with confidence. A few minor defects should not affect the major conclusions. However, evidence of powerful selection, including substantial non-response, will mean that the findings cannot be generalised.

The complete list for the appraisal of surveys

The essential questions

Who was studied?
How was the sample obtained?
What was the response rate?

The detailed questions★

Design

Are the aims clearly stated?
Is the design appropriate to the stated objectives?
Was the sample size justified?
Are the measurements likely to be valid and reliable?
Are the statistical methods described?
Is there a suggestion of haste?

Conduct

Did untoward events occur during the study?

Analysis

Were the basic data adequately described?
Do the numbers add up?
Was the statistical significance assessed?
Were the findings serendipitous?

Interpretation

What do the main findings mean?
How could selection bias arise?
How are null findings interpreted?
Are important effects overlooked?
Can the results be generalised?
How do the results compare with previous reports?
What implications does the study have for your practice?

★ The questions in italics are the standard ones which were described in Chapter 6.

8 Appraising cohort studies

This chapter presents the issues which are relevant primarily to cohort studies. These are arranged in two parts: the brief essential questions and the more detailed specific questions. An explanation is given for each item. These lists are then combined, at the end of the chapter, with the list of standard questions described in Chapter 6. These lists provide a complete guide to the appraisal of cohort studies.

The essential questions

Cohort studies follow patients through time to determine what becomes of them. The object may be to follow the natural time course of disease, or to determine whether some medical intervention has had an unintended consequence. Thus, the appraisal of cohort studies focuses on the patient group and the outcome being investigated, asking:

Who exactly has been studied?
Was a control group used? Should one have been used?
How adequate was the follow-up?

The specific questions

The specific questions extend the concern with the nature of the study group and the details of the follow-up. They also explore the factors which can contribute to misleading findings.

Is the design appropriate to the stated aims?
Was the exposure/intervention accurately measured?

Were relevant outcome measures ignored?
Did the analysis allow for the passage of time?
What else might influence the observed outcome?

Rationale for the essential questions

Who exactly has been studied?

The features of the group being studied are important because the events which befall patients depend crucially on their characteristics. The nature and number of clinical events which occur among patients will depend on the duration and severity of their illness, the range of interventions to which they have been exposed, and the presence or absence of other medical conditions. Thus, the key to interpreting the findings is a clear idea of who has been studied, enabling the reader to ask: is this a surprising result? The extent to which the findings can be generalised to other groups of patients will also depend on who has been studied. Thus, the source of the patients should be specified, for example, whether they have been identified through a specialist clinic or through general practice. The definition of eligibility for entry to the study, such as the disease definition or the nature of the exposure, should be given. Finally, if the study subjects have been obtained by some form of sampling (for example, selecting GPs and taking a sample of their patients) the details of this should be reviewed. These will indicate whether the sample obtained is likely to be representative of a wider group.

Was a control group used? Should one have been used?

Follow-up studies investigating exposure/intervention cannot easily be interpreted when data have been collected only on the exposed group. Suppose that the cancer risk of industrial pollution were being assessed. Cancers occur spontaneously, so the true question is whether there is an increase in the frequency of cancer among those exposed. This can be determined only by comparison with some control group who resemble the study group in all ways except exposure. A crucial question concerns the appropriateness of the control group: does it enable a fair comparison to be made?

How adequate was the follow-up?

In follow-up studies patients have many opportunities to disappear. Marriage, death, emigration, or admission to a long-stay hospital can all result in patients being lost to follow-up. Whatever the reasons for it, those lost to follow-up are likely to differ from those who remain in view. The greater the extent of this loss the greater the potential for bias. Thus, the key questions are: how great was the loss? And to what extent, given the circumstances of the study, could this influence the results?

Another crucial aspect of follow-up is the way that the outcome was measured. For signal events like death or the diagnosis of cancer, measurement is straightforward because the information will be stated in official records. Physiological or biochemical measures of disease status, such as peak flow for respiratory disease or plasma creatinine for renal disease, also provide objective measures. But when clinical judgement is being used, for example to arrive at a diagnosis, there is an opportunity for error. Equally, when patients are being interviewed, the nature of the questioning, either probing or passing on, could influence the answers obtained. Thus, the question to be asked is: could the method of obtaining the outcome data materially affect the result? It is important then that the person taking these decisions is blind to the exposure group, otherwise bias might occur.

Finally, the length of follow-up should be reviewed to clarify whether it was long enough to have a reasonable chance of detecting important events. This is particularly important for studies in which no events were observed. The minimum length of follow-up depends on the events being studied. For example, if the study investigated pain and discomfort after discharge from day-case surgery, then a few weeks of follow-up would be sufficient. However, if the aim was to detect adverse events associated with a new treatment then a much longer follow-up would be required. Side-effects may take several months to develop. Further, if there was interest in diseases like cancer, which can take many years to occur, then a substantially longer follow-up would be needed. The question to be asked is: how long could it be until the events of interest occur? The follow-up period should be substantially longer than the expected time.

Rationale for the specific questions

Is the design appropriate to the stated aims?
Was the exposure/intervention accurately measured?
Were relevant outcome measures ignored?
What else might influence the observed outcome?

Did the analysis allow for the passage of time?
Are the findings unexpected?

Is the design appropriate to the stated aims?

Cohort studies are used to answer questions of the form "What happens next?". They are clearly the method of choice when studying disease prognosis, but they are also used for investigating consequences of exposure to potentially harmful agents. Cohort studies are commonly used to investigate causality – for example, whether an exposure caused a particular disease. However, they are not the best method for answering this question: a clinical trial would be preferred. However, it is plainly unethical to expose people to potentially noxious agents in a clinical trial. Cohort studies are used instead, recognising their limitations.

One area in which cohort studies are particularly poor is the assessment of treatment efficacy. It is often possible to identify cohorts of patients who received different treatments, and it might appear tempting to compare outcomes. For example, the outcome for those receiving radical surgery could be compared with that for patients with the same condition who were more conservatively treated. The problem is that there will often be good clinical reasons for the choice of operation: perhaps those with the more serious disease receive the more radical treatment. Whatever the basis for choice, the two groups being compared are likely to be different before they are treated. Differences in outcome cannot then be assigned to the nature of the treatment; they could easily be due to the way patients were allocated to each treatment.

Was the exposure/intervention accurately measured?

When the cohort study is investigating the consequences of some medical intervention or exposure to a noxious chemical, the nature of the exposure/intervention should be properly described. It is best if the extent of exposure has been measured objectively. For example, the amount of exposure to medical X-rays could be obtained through case-note searches of the type and number of X-rays that each patient had had. It would also be possible to confirm that the controls had not been exposed.

Sometimes the exposure will be more difficult to quantify – for example, exposure to an environmental hazard such as airborne pollution from an industrial plant. Residence close to the plant could be used as a proxy for exposure, but individuals will vary in the amounts of time they spend at home. Further, some of the control group, chosen because they live far from the plant, could actually work at the plant. Measuring exposure can be difficult, especially if the concern is with chronic exposure, when individuals' exposure levels can change over time. Thus, whenever exposure/intervention is described, two key questions to be asked are "How accurately was exposure measured" and "Could some of the controls have been exposed?".

Were relevant outcome measures ignored?

The impact of medical interventions or exposure to noxious agents could be measured in different ways. For example, if an atmospheric pollutant is suspected of causing or exacerbating asthma, exposed individuals could be followed up in several ways. Deaths from asthma might not be helpful because they would be rare, but emergency hospital admissions for asthma could well be used. Alternatively, outcome could be assessed in general practice, counting recorded new diagnoses or exacerbations of asthma. Even indirect measures, such as requests for anti-asthma medication, or the cashing of prescriptions, could be used. Finally, a community survey could be carried out to investigate symptoms of breathlessness or wheezing. The different outcome measures vary not just in their frequency but also in their severity and their validity. Published papers should give some rationale for their choice of outcome measure, but it is up to the reader to decide how best the outcome could have been assessed.

Did the analysis allow for the passage of time?

If cohort studies follow people for several years they may need to allow for the ageing of study participants. Most diseases increase in frequency with age so the analysis should take account of this. Further, if important factors which could influence the outcome have been identified these should also be incorporated into the analysis. It can be difficult for the non-statistician to be sure whether the methods are truly appropriate, but it will be possible to check that some attempts have been made to cope with the complexities which have been identified.

What else might influence the outcome?

The major limitation of cohort studies is that the researcher has no control over the group to be investigated. The study group is selected because they have some disease or have been exposed to some potentially noxious agent. Individuals who develop a disease may differ in many ways from those who are disease-free. Equally, those who have been exposed to a noxious agent are likely to differ from those who have not. The process of selecting individuals with some defined characteristic can influence the study outcome. Thus, the outcome needs to be reviewed to determine which factors, clinical and behavioural, could influence it. These could be aspects of individual behaviour, such as smoking, drinking, diet, and exercise, or characteristics of the disease or its management. Having identified these factors, the paper can be inspected to see whether these factors were investigated and, if so, how they were allowed for in the analysis.

The complete list for the appraisal of cohort studies

The essential questions

Who exactly has been studied?
Was a control group used? Should one have been used?
How adequate was the follow-up?

The detailed questions*

Design

Are the aims clearly stated?
Is the design appropriate to the stated aims?
Was the sample size justified?
Are the measurements likely to be valid and reliable?
Was the exposure/intervention accurately measured?
Were relevant outcome measures ignored?
Are the statistical methods described?

Conduct

Did untoward events occur during the study?

Analysis

Did the analysis allow for the passage of time?
Do the numbers add up?
Were the basic data adequately described?
Was statistical significance assessed?

Interpretation

What do the main findings mean?
What else might influence the observed outcome?
How are null findings interpreted?
Are important effects overlooked?
How do the results compare with previous reports?
What implications does the study have for your practice?

* The questions in italics are the standard ones which were described in Chapter 6.

9 Appraising clinical trials

This chapter presents the issues which are relevant primarily to clinical trials. These are arranged in two parts: the brief essential questions and the more detailed specific questions. An explanation is given for each item. These lists are then combined, at the end of the chapter, with the list of standard questions described in Chapter 6. These lists provide a complete guide to the appraisal of clinical trials.

The essential questions

Clinical trials are the method for assessing the effectiveness of specific treatments. In essence they involve comparing one treatment with another to determine which is better. The key requirement for clinical trials is that a fair comparison is made. The essential appraisal questions are directed at the main reasons why the comparison might not be fair:

Were treatments randomly allocated?
Were all the patients accounted for?
Were outcomes assessed blind?

The specific questions

The specific questions also search for potential causes of unfairness in the comparison of treatments. However, they extend the evaluation into other areas and inspect the overall quality of the trial. Evidence of poor quality can cast doubt on a study, even when the brief appraisal suggests that the comparison appears to be fair. The questions also review the wider significance of the findings.

The extent to which the findings can be generalised depends on how the study was conducted: the types of patients, the nature of the treatment, and the way the outcome was assessed.

Could the choice of subjects influence the size of treatment effect?
How was the randomisation carried out?
Were there ambiguities in the description of the treatment and its administration?
Could lack of blinding introduce bias?
Are the outcomes clinically relevant?
Were the treatment groups comparable at baseline?
Were deviations from planned treatment reported?
Were results analysed by intention to treat?
Is the size of effect clinically important?
Were side-effects reported?

Rationale for the essential questions

Were treatments randomly allocated?

For a fair comparison the two treatments must be given to similar types of patients. This can be best achieved by randomly allocating patients to one of the two treatments. (The process uses computer-generated random numbers to avoid any problems of human frailty.) If randomisation has not been used, the patients receiving the two treatments are likely to be systematically different. The term 'quasi-randomised' is a warning signal; it usually means that patients have been allocated to treatments using a method which is convenient to the researchers (for example, by day of the week). But the convenience may result in subtle differences between the two groups.

Were all the patients accounted for?

In clinical studies contact with some patients may be lost. The concern in clinical trials is whether the patients who disappear are special in any way. For example, patients may fail to attend a scheduled appointment because they are so severely ill that they are unable to travel. Alternatively, they may be completely recovered, and not see any need to attend. If one of the treatments being tested was truly effective then patients who were being cured might not attend. If the other treatment was much less effective it might well be the very sick who do not attend. It is not possible to know why some patients disappear from follow-up. However, doubts about the fairness of the comparison emerge if a substantial number of those who were randomised have disappeared. Concern is particularly heightened if more patients are lost from one treatment group than the other.

Were outcomes assessed blind?

When clinical judgement is needed to assess the outcome of treatment there is the opportunity for personal views to intrude. One researcher may be an enthusiast for a new treatment, and may subconsciously record a better outcome for the patients receiving it. Another researcher, aware of this possible bias, may over-compensate and give a better rating to the other treatment. The problem is prevented if those assessing treatment outcome are blind to the treatment each patient received.

Rationale for the specific questions

Could the choice of subjects influence the size of treatment effect?

To be able to assess the effects of a treatment the source and nature of the patients studied need to be fully described. It is possible that a treatment which is highly effective for the severely ill patients seen at a specialist centre would have little impact on those with a milder form of the disease who are managed by a general practitioner. The information which should be given is:

- The setting from which the patients were recruited (community, hospital, or specialist clinic)
- The diagnostic criteria for entry to the trial
- Factors which led to patients being excluded from the study (for example, contra-indications to therapy)
- A description of the duration and severity of disease at entry to the study

This information allows the reader to decide the extent to which the study findings apply elsewhere. In particular, it helps to answer the question "Could this treatment help my patients?".

How was the randomisation carried out?

The randomisation of patients should be organised so as to minimise the opportunities for the randomisation code to be broken. Thus, the report should indicate how the process was undertaken. In the past the randomisation codes were sometimes held in individually sealed envelopes, but nowadays the codes are usually kept at a remote central trial office. As each patient is entered the clinician would phone the trial office to be told the appropriate code. For example, in a drugs trial the two treatments might be identically packaged, one labelled A the other B. The clinician would be given the appropriate letter for each patient, thus preserving blindness to treatment group.

Were there ambiguities in the description of the treatment and its administration?

To be used in practice the treatments tested in a clinical trial need to be fully described. If the information is absent, it may be difficult for others to use a successful treatment in their own practice. Further, if these details have not been clearly worked out the treatment may not have been given properly to all the study patients. Were this to happen the size of any treatment effect could be reduced.

Could lack of blinding introduce bias?

Bias can be introduced in several ways when it is known which treatment each patient received. It is better that everyone – patient, clinician and statistician – be blind to treatment details. Patients who believe they are getting an expensive new drug may report being better than they really are. There is evidence that, through mechanisms which are little understood, these patients may actually experience clinical benefit.

The management given to patients by the caring physician could also be affected by knowledge of the treatment. If one treatment is thought to be less effective, those given it might receive more care and attention to compensate for the anticipated deficiencies. If knowledge of the treatment group influences overall management, bias could result.

The question of biased outcome assessment was discussed in the brief appraisal, although bias during the statistical analysis was not. If it were known which treatment group was which, there could be a temptation to search the data for some difference which would support one of the therapies. Obscure differences which did not support this therapy might be disregarded and only supportive ones reported. If there appears to be some data-torturing, be suspicious if the analysis was not carried out blind to treatment group.

Are the outcomes clinically relevant?

Deciding whether a treatment is effective is not always easy. For some diseases there may be an obvious yardstick: for example, for cancer it might be the length of time for which patients survive. For other diseases, such as rheumatism, clear-cut measures such as time to death are not appropriate. Alternative measures, such as levels of disease activity, extent of disease-related physical mobility, or quality of life, need to be used. There are often many different ways in which the effect of treatment could be measured. It is always worth asking whether the one which was used provides the best way to assess the management of this disease. At its most extreme, the treatment might improve one aspect of the disease (level of symptoms or patient satisfaction) while other aspects deteriorate (leading to serious complications or even death). Short-term measures (for example, patient status at 2 weeks) are particularly suspect.

When several outcomes measures have been used, it is best if one of them has been nominated as the primary measure to be used to judge treatment. This guards against the dangers of multiple testing, when out of a host of measures the one producing (spurious) statistical significance is highlighted while the others are overlooked.

Were the treatment groups comparable at baseline?

Random allocation of treatments is used to guard against bias in assigning patients to treatments. However, this technique does not guarantee that the two treatment groups will be identical at the start of the study. By the play of chance it is possible for more of the severely ill patients to be allocated to one of the groups than the other. Thus, the two groups need to be assessed to determine whether they were similar at the start of the study. This evaluation should focus on those items most relevant to prognosis and outcome. For example, suppose an antihypertensive drug were being tested and effectiveness were being measured by the number of patients who had a stroke or a heart attack. Age, gender, serum cholesterol, and cigarette smoking are major risk factors for these diseases, so it would be important to check that the two groups were similar for these factors.

If there are differences at baseline in important factors, this need not negate the whole study. Careful statistical analysis can go a long way to take account of such differences. Thus, when they exist, the question is whether they have been allowed for in the analysis.

Were deviations from planned treatment reported?

Several events can affect the smooth running of a trial. Patients may fail to comply with therapy. They may have their treatments stopped, because of side-effects or concerns about a deteriorating condition. They may be transferred to other therapies or may be given additional treatments to those under investigation. If any of these events were to happen more commonly in one group than in the other, a fair comparison could not be made. Managing one group differently to the other could produce a difference in outcome unrelated to the treatments being studied. Good trials report these details separately for the two treatment groups, allowing the reader to assess the potential for bias. Studies which do not report these details arouse suspicion.

Were results analysed by intention to treat?

In the course of the trial patients may have their treatments changed and may even swap from one treatment to the other. Whatever has happened, the best advice is to analyse the study by the groups to which the patients were first allocated. The concern is that patients who change treatments, or even withdraw from the study, may be systematically different to those who do not change. Excluding these patients from the analysis could introduce differences between the two groups of patients at entry into the study. The comparison of treatments would no longer be fair. (It might be argued that bias could arise because some patients had their treatment changed. This could occur, but it is considered a lesser evil than excluding these patients.)

Were side-effects reported?

Many treatments have unwanted side-effects: amoxycillin can cause nausea and diarrhoea; amitriptyline causes dry mouth and sedation; and surgical operations certainly have their hazards. Thus, the beneficial effect of any therapy has to be balanced against its side-effects. Often the balance is clear, when the therapeutic effect outweighs the adverse effects. But when two similar treatments are being compared, a difference in side-effect profile could be more important than a treatment difference.

The complete list for the appraisal of clinical trials

The essential questions
Were treatments randomly allocated?
Were all the patients accounted for?
Were outcomes assessed blind?

The detailed questions*

Design
Are the aims clearly stated?
Was the sample size justified?
Are the measurements likely to be valid and reliable?
Could the choice of subjects influence the size of treatment effect?
Were there ambiguities in the description of the treatment and its administration?
Are the statistical methods described?
Could lack of blinding introduce bias?
Are the outcomes clinically relevant?

Conduct
How was the randomisation carried out?
Did untoward events occur during the study?

Analysis
Were the treatment groups comparable at baseline?
Were results analysed by intention to treat?
Was the statistical significance assessed?
Were the basic data adequately described?
Do the numbers add up?
Were side-effects reported?

Interpretation
What do the main findings mean?
How are null findings interpreted?
Are important effects overlooked?
How do the results compare with previous reports?
What implications does the study have for your practice?

---

* The questions in italics are the standard ones which were described in Chapter 6.

10 Appraising case–control studies

This chapter presents the issues which are relevant primarily to case–control studies. These are arranged in two parts: the brief essential questions and the more detailed specific questions. An explanation is given for each item. These lists are then combined, at the end of the chapter, with the list of standard questions described in Chapter 6. These lists provide a complete guide to the appraisal of case–control studies.

The essential questions

Case–control studies investigate why certain people develop a specific illness. They can also investigate why some sets of patients behave as they do – for example, why some do not attend for cervical screening. The studies seek out the factors which mark out these individuals as being special, in the hope that this will identify the causes of the disease or the explanation for their behaviour. The method does this by comparing the characteristics of those with a disease (or characteristic of interest) against a suitable group of control individuals. The assumption is that differences between cases and controls will reveal why cases become cases. The essential questions focus on the validity of this assumption.

How were the cases obtained?
Is the control group appropriate?
Were data collected the same way for cases and controls?

The specific questions

The specific questions are also concerned with the interpretation of the case and control comparisons, but they deal with the methodological problems which are particularly acute for case–control studies.

Is the design appropriate to the aims?
Where are the biases?
Could there be confounding?
Was there data-dredging?

Rationale for the essential questions

How were the cases obtained?

The characteristics of the cases should be clearly stated. This would include the definition of a case which should be broad enough to ensure that true cases are not missed, yet specific enough to ensure that only true cases are included. In many instances the case definition will be a statement of diagnostic criteria for the disease together with any exclusion criteria (such as concomitant disease).

The source of the cases should also be given whether from the general population or some specialist centre. The average severity of the condition is likely to vary with the source of the cases. Another concern is whether the cases represent newly diagnosed disease, or whether they are cases with long-standing illness. Those with long-standing disease are a selected group; those who have been cured or have died will be lost. Selective loss could bias the severity of the disease in two ways: those cured may have had mild disease, whereas those who died might have had more severe illness. Bias could also arise if some of those who were sought for the study were not included in it. Patients who avoid inclusion in research studies tend to differ from those included.

These details of the cases studied are central to the interpretation of the results. Atypical cases can produce atypical findings, so that the nature of the cases will also influence the extent to which the findings can be generalised.

Is the control group appropriate?

Selecting appropriate controls is one of the major challenges of case–control studies. They are generally selected from the same source as the cases, be that the community, general practice or specialist centre. The intention is that they should resemble the cases, except that they do not have the disease being studied. Since there are many forces of selection which determine where cases are managed, it is best if both cases and controls have been subject to the same forces. Controls are usually selected to be similar in terms of age, sex, social class, and area of residence to the cases.

The obsession with the comparability of controls follows from the analysis of these studies: evidence about causes of disease comes from a comparison of cases and controls. If differing forces of selection introduce differences between cases and controls, these might be mistaken for risk factors for the disease.

Were data collected in the same way for cases and controls?

Having recruited cases and controls, both must be asked about past exposure to potential risk factors. This information should be obtained in the same way for each, whether by interview, postal questionnaire or case-note review. But even using the same method may not produce identical information gathering. If the data collector knows which are cases and which controls, then interviews or case-note searches may be influenced. Blinding to case control status should be used where possible.

Another source of problems is recall bias: patients who have a serious disease tend to review their past history in detail to find an explanation for their illness. Thus they are more likely to report events which the controls might forget. Case–control studies are bedevilled by biased information gathering. The details of the data-collection techniques need to be scrutinised carefully to determine whether data collection was identical for cases and controls.

Rationale for the specific questions

Is the design appropriate to the aims?

Case–control studies are a powerful research method, but they have limitations. They involve collecting data retrospectively, after cases have developed the disease (or other characteristics of interest). They cannot be used to assess the effectiveness of a new treatment. They are often used to investigate possible cause and effect: whether a specific factor is associated with the risk of developing a disease. However, they seldom provide definitive evidence for cause and effect because of their potential for bias. Finally, because the cases are often highly selected, they cannot be used to make more general statements about how common certain features occur: this would require a survey.

Where are the biases?

Case–control studies are notorious for their susceptibility to bias. The brief appraisal questions introduced the idea that bias could arise through the selection of cases and controls and through the method of data collection. But there are many subtle variants on these biases. One form of this is surveillance bias; individuals who are taking regular medication will be more likely to have regular contact with doctors. Thus, newly occurring asymptomatic or mild diseases are more likely to be diagnosed. This could create an apparent but spurious relationship between the medication and the new mild disease.

Another form of bias is misclassification bias: some of the cases may not have the disease of interest but suffer instead from a condition which resembles it. For example, endometrial hyperplasia could be misclassified as frank carcinoma. Then any factors associated with hyperplasia (for example, exogenous oestrogens) would be falsely associated with the cancer.

The willingness of patients to participate in studies and provide information can also result in bias. Those who have a serious illness are likely to differ on both counts from other groups in the community. In short, the opportunities for bias in case–control studies are legion. The challenge is to identify the source and to try to estimate what effect it could have on the study findings. Whenever associations between diseases and risk factors are identified these should be reviewed by asking "How else could this have occurred?", "What might be special about the cases?" and "How could the measurements be biased?". Case–control studies should always be approached in the expectation that there will be bias.

Could there be confounding?

Confounding arises when an observed association between two variables is due to the action of a third factor. For example, excess sugar consumption will lead to an increase in dental caries. It will also increase the risk of developing mature-onset diabetes. There could thus be an apparent relationship between caries and diabetes which would arise because some individuals had a particular fondness for sugar.

Case–control studies are often used to investigate why disease occurs in certain individuals. Thus, whenever a case–control shows that a disease is related to some factor, attention should be given to other factors that both might be related to. Could a third factor be driving the observed relationship? It is often difficult to guess what the third factor might be, but the subject should be raised at some point in the discussion section. When confounding factors are identified in a study they should be taken into account in the analysis. There are standard statistical methods to do this. It can be difficult to tell whether these have been used correctly, but at least they should have been used.

Was there data-dredging?

Case–control studies are often exploratory, casting a wide net to see what can be caught. These studies are asking why cases are different from controls (i.e. what is it that is special about cases?). They allow a number of different hypotheses to be tested at the same time. Data are collected on as many different items as the imagination and resources of the researchers allow. The analysis then involves trawling through the variables, looking for anything of interest. When this is done, multiple significance testing becomes a major hazard. Calculated P-values can no longer be interpreted at face value, and some instances of spurious statistical significance should be expected. Thus, reports should be carefully scrutinised for evidence of multiple testing, and findings interpreted more cautiously if this has occurred.

The complete list for the appraisal of case–control studies

The essential questions

How were the cases obtained?
Is the control group appropriate?
Were data collected the same way for cases and controls?

The detailed questions*

Design

Are the aims clearly stated?
Is the method appropriate to the aims?
Was the sample size justified?
Are the measurements likely to be valid and reliable?
Are the statistical methods described?

Conduct

Did untoward events occur during the study?

Analysis

Were the basic data adequately described?
Do the numbers add up?
Was there data-dredging?
as the statistical significance assessed?

Interpretation

What do the main findings mean?
Where are the biases?
Could there be confounding?
How are null findings interpreted?
Are important effects overlooked?
How do the results compare with previous reports?
What implications does the study have for your practice?

---

* The questions in italics are the standard ones which were described in Chapter 6.

11 Appraising review papers

This chapter presents the issues which are relevant primarily to review papers and meta-analyses. These are arranged in two parts: the brief essential questions and the more detailed specific questions. An explanation is given for each item. These lists are then combined, at the end of the chapter, with those items from the list of standard questions which are relevant to this type of study. These lists provide a complete guide to the appraisal of review papers and meta-analyses.

The essential questions

Preparing a review of published research calls for the same diligence and rigour which characterises the best of original research. Systematic reviews are heir to the same pitfalls and biases as original research. Thus, it is little surprise that the appraisal of review papers follows an identical sequence to that used for the research methods, focusing in turn on the design, the conduct of the study, and the analysis of the review materials.

How were the papers identified?
How was the quality of papers assessed?
How were the results summarised?

The specific questions

The specific questions explore in more detail how the study was conducted, to see how the pitfalls common to review papers were dealt with.

Is the topic well defined?
Was publication bias taken into account?
Was missing information sought?
Were the detailed study designs reviewed?
Was heterogeneity of effect investigated?
Are there other findings which merit attention?
Are the conclusions justified?

Rationale for the essential questions

How were the papers identified?

Research papers are the raw data of a review and need to be gathered with care. In the past some review articles were prepared using the personal set of papers which their author had collected over the years. These will reflect the interests of the author and are likely to be incomplete. The concern is that they may be a biased sample of all papers. Computerised searches are so easy to conduct that they are now essential for any good review. The details of the search should be described: which databases were searched, and what key terms were used in the search. But even computerised searches will not yield all relevant reports. Because of the way papers are indexed in the databases, some papers will not be found even when all the sensible key terms have been used in the search. Thus, to be complete, manual searches of selected journals need to be undertaken. Plainly, the workload of these searches will be so large that they will be possible only if special funding is provided. The absence of these extended systematic searches should temper the conclusions which can be drawn from a review.

One consequence of exhaustive searching is that a large number of possibly relevant studies will be identified. Clearly defined criteria will be needed to decide which to include in the review, because they are particularly pertinent to the topic, and which to exclude. These criteria would need to be inspected carefully, to determine whether they might bias the papers to be included.

How was the quality of papers assessed?

Not all research studies are well designed and conducted. Including studies of poor quality on the same footing as those of high quality is plainly undesirable. Thus, the quality of the papers identified needs to be assessed. This can be achieved with formal check lists, such as those presented in this book. Subjective assessment of quality, in the absence of a list of specific points, is less satisfactory.

The strength of evidence from a paper also depends on the research method which was used. Controlled clinical trials are reckoned to provide the most powerful evidence followed in decreasing order of strength by cohort studies, case–control studies, surveys, and case-series. The assessment of quality and strength of evidence is an essential prelude to summarising the results from the papers identified.

How were the results summarised?

The results of the individual studies can be presented in a table or figure to allow the reader to judge whether, on balance, they give a consistent answer. This display will also indicate the amount of variation between individual studies. Individual judgement can be used to draw conclusions from the data. But far better is to use the statistical methods of meta-analysis. The major advantage of systematic reviews is that, by combining studies, they have substantially increased power to detect significant results. This power can be harnessed only by using the appropriate statistical techniques.

One unanswered question is what to do with poor-quality studies. Excluding them entirely could be wasteful of information. One solution is to use a weighting system where the poor studies are given such a low weight that they have only a small effect on the conclusions (the details of these weighting systems are described in standard texts on meta-analysis). An alternative approach is to conduct what are called sensitivity analyses. This involves first summarising the results with all possible studies included. Then, those of the lowest quality would be excluded and the analysis repeated. This process would be repeated, progressively higher quality thresholds being set for papers to be included. This would indicate how sensitive the conclusions are to the inclusion of poor-quality papers. If broadly the same result is obtained across a range of quality thresholds then the findings can be accepted.

Rationale for the specific questions

Is the topic well defined?

The focus of the review should be clearly stated. The review is more likely to identify all relevant articles when limited to a narrow area of medicine. Wide-ranging reviews, for example covering the diagnosis, treatment, long-term prognosis and epidemiology, may well miss important papers. Such broad overviews have their place in research, but they tend to present the personal view of the author. They should be distinguished from the exhaustive process of producing a systematic review.

Were the detailed study designs reviewed?

Individual studies often vary in the details of their design – for example, in the types of patient they have studied (diagnostic criteria, age range etc.) or in the ways in which treatment was given (dosage level, timing of treatments etc.). These differences should be identified and compared with the size of effects which were reported. Broadly similar findings across a range of clinical conditions do not just strengthen the conclusions, they indicate that the findings can be more widely generalised.

Was missing information sought?

Sometimes information on some key details about a study is not contained in the published report. This could make it difficult to assess the quality of a study or, in some instances, to interpret the results. Painstaking reviewers will write to the authors requesting these details.

Was publication bias taken into account?

Papers which report positive findings have a higher chance of publication than those which conclude that a new treatment was ineffective or a hoped-for effect was not found. This may reflect the enthusiasm with which researchers seek publication, or the reluctance of journals to accept negative reports. The concern about unpublished studies is that their findings might be systematically different from those that were published. If included in the review, these studies might weight the findings sufficiently to lead to quite different conclusions.

Finding unpublished studies is difficult. It could involve writing to researchers known to be active in the field, asking whether they have conducted, or possibly know of, unpublished studies. Details of any studies uncovered would then have to be sought. When some effort has been made to find them, more weight can be given to the conclusions from the review. When unpublished papers have not been sought, the main findings may be biased – they most likely overestimate the sizes of any effects. The degree of overestimation can only be guessed at, so the only safe advice is to interpret with caution.

Was heterogeneity of effect investigated?

Some variation in results of individual studies would be expected just by the play of chance. However, heterogeneity of effect can occur because of differences in design. Formal statistical methods should be used to determine whether the amount of variation is greater than would be expected by chance. If this has occurred it should be investigated further to see which of the design features might explain it. For example, if there were large differences in the ages of the patients investigated, then individual studies could be subdivided by age to see whether the effect is consistent within age groups.

Even if there is no statistical evidence of heterogeneity, the studies should still be inspected carefully to see whether studies which share design features have broadly similar results. (Unfortunately the statistical tests are rather poor at detecting heterogeneity.) It might be, for example, that large effects are seen among the young with more modest effects among the elderly. Whenever there is evidence of heterogeneity, the process summarising all the studies with a single measure becomes doubtful.

Are there other findings which merit attention?

Systematic reviews are a major undertaking, so that their results should be inspected with great care. They should contain all the valid studies on a particular topic. They will clarify not only what is known but also what is not yet known: they should cast in sharp relief the gaps in current knowledge. This will help to identify the major research questions in the field which are yet to be answered.

Are the conclusions justified?

The interpretation of systematic reviews is as prone to errors as is the interpretation of any data. Thus, the reader should ask: Do they reflect the weight of evidence? Was due allowance made for the strengths of the research methods? Were defects in the studies taken into account? Review articles may appear unchallengeable, particularly those which have involved extensive searches and have combined findings using meta-analysis techniques. This semblance of infallibility should be rejected; review articles are prepared by people, and people make mistakes. As for any other research method, readers should make up their own minds about the conclusions.

The complete list for the appraisal of review papers

The essential questions

How were the papers identified?
How was the quality of papers assessed?
How were the results summarised?

The detailed questions*

Design

Is the topic well defined?
Are the statistical methods described?

Conduct

Were the detailed study designs reviewed?
Was missing information sought?

Analysis

Were the basic data adequately described?
Was publication bias taken into account?
Was heterogeneity of effect investigated?

Interpretation

What do the main findings mean?
Are there other findings which merit attention?
Are the conclusions justified?
How do the findings compare with previous reports?
What implications does the study have for your practice?

* The questions in italics are the standard ones which were described in Chapter 6.

Index